AUTOPHAGY

*UNLOCK YOUR BODY'S NATURAL
CELLULAR REPAIR CODE FOR WEIGHT
LOSS, ANTI-AGING, ENHANCED HEALTH
AND REVITALIZATION BENEFITS*

Michael D Kaiser

<u>Published By:</u>

Clinic Network

P.O. Box 1801

Mentor, OH 44060

<u>Legal Disclaimer:</u>

Table of Contents

Introduction

The term "Autophagy" comes from the Greek word "self-eating"—and that is its function. It is a normal process inside every one of our cells where whole organelles, that are destroyed, or not serving any function, are broken down and any individual components produced in the process are recycled as a source of energy. This process usually takes place on a basal level to guarantee the quality and survival of cells. It is the cellular equivalent to "taking out the trash", the only difference is that if we don't take out the trash we still continue to live our lives, whereas our cells cannot. Autophagy can be both, pro-survival and post-death, so it is critical that we don't hold it for long and commit our lives to have it stimulated at all times.

That said, this book will take you through a step by step method to learn how you can take advantage of autophagy. You will learn how you can unlock your body's natural cellular repair code for weight loss, anti-aging, and acquire the health benefits of autophagy. Keep reading to learn more.

Chapter 1: Getting Started with Autophagy

In Greek, autophagy means to eat one's self. Simply put, autophagy is the mechanism of the body to clean out damaged cells, in order to redevelop newer, healthier cells.

"Auto" means self while "phagy" means eat. And that is how the literal meaning "self-eating" originates from.

But how can cannibalistic be the next trend in general body health? And how can it be a digestive phase we need to try and implement into our systems? The answer depends on the primitive nature of the human body.

The body can realize a lot of things when subjected to positive stress.

When we were hunters and gatherers, the human body was not aware of the time when it would get its next meal. So it switched into a state of stress and completed natural cleansing after hours of consuming food.

During this period, the body acquired dangerous and damaged cells. These cells could cause destruction in the form of cancer.

According to the US National Library of Medicine National Institute of Health, the ritual of acquiring three square meals per day plus snacks in between isn't a natural, evolutionary behavior that helps the body in any way.

The study shows that in a sixteen-hour fasting period, the body triggers "mechanisms that involve a metabolic change to fat metabolism and ketone production, and stimulation of adaptive cellular stress responses that repair and prevent molecular damage."

But, how can we implement autophagy and body cleansing into our normal schedules?

Understanding the General Benefit
to Your Health

Intermittent fasting, body cleansing, and autophagy are terms used to refer to the body's natural process of exfoliating the body from the inside out. The greatest benefit of body cleansing is permitting your body to naturally reduce the oxidative stress that occurs from everyday living. This generally affects the aging process.

The best thing about this process is that you don't need to adhere to a fasting diet forever to experience the benefits of allowing your body to follow a cycle of cellular cleansing.

Some people decide to adhere to a normal routine of consuming 1-2 full nutritious meals per day. This provides their bodies with 6-16 hours of daily cleansing. Some select a 24-hour weekly cleansing or even a 48-hour monthly cleansing.

The timing is left to you to select what you think works for your body. Providing your body with a natural restart without implementing regular cleansing can lead to a long list of health benefits. These comprise of prevention of liver disease, cancer, autoimmune diseases, and diabetes.

Autophagy is receiving a lot of focus for the role it may play in cancer treatment. It declines as we age, and this means cells that fail to work, or may cause harm are allowed to multiply, which the MO of cancer cells.

Although all cancer begins from some form of defective cells, the body should detect and remove those cells using the autophagy process. That is the reason why some researchers continue to concentrate on the possibility that autophagy may decrease the risk of cancer.

The Mechanism of Autophagy

Autophagy in eukaryotes has three different channels, namely micro-autophagy, macro-autophagy, and chaperone-mediated autophagy. While all the three separate pathways result in the lysosomal degradation of cellular cargo, macro-autophagy is the most studied.

The mechanism of macro-autophagy is ingrained among eukaryotes and is defined by the encapsulation of cellular cargo within the double-membrane vesicles known as autophagosomes.

In the yeast, the development of autophagosomes near the targeted cargo is achieved by autophagy-related proteins that are admitted hierarchically to the phagophore assembly site(PAS).

At the PAS, the protein activator complexes support the de novo development of a double membrane structure known as phagophore, the lipid components for which are extracted from the Golgi-endosome system.

In mammals, the special PAS-like structure is yet to be chosen, numerous cellular organelles, including the plasma membrane, are considered to work as origins for the assembly of a phagophore. Once other Atg proteins are admitted, the isolation membrane is extended into a phagophore, which finally integrates at the free end to create an autophagosome that surrounds the cargo.

Once they are created, the autophagosomes go through a maturation process as they are carried along the endocytic pathway before joining with the lysosomes to create autophagolysosomes. The cellular cargo transported by the autophagosomes are finally degraded by the hydrolytic enzymes of the lysosomes and the degradation products are carried to the cytoplasm for cell use.

The remaining autophagy pathways do not need the details of autophagosomes. When it comes to microautophagy, the lysosome directly surrounds portions of the cytoplasm while in chaperone-mediated autophagy; the individual chaperone proteins connect to the cargo and transfer it across the lysosomal membrane for degradation.

How Long Until Autophagy Starts

If you want to learn how long until autophagy kicks in, then this section is right for you.

Autophagy Regulators

Autophagy is a metabolic process that converts cellular debris and dysfunctional organelles into energy via self-eating. It is activated through specific metabolic pathways like AMPK, reactive oxygen species, and things such as calcium, Nf-kb, and many more.

While there is little to learn about autophagy, the existing research indicates that most of the signaling takes place via the pathways of AMPK and Mtor.

- Mtor is known as the *Mammalian Target of Rapamycin.* It is the body's master nutrient controller that impacts cellular growth, synthesis of protein, and anabolism. It increases the activation of insulin receptors and the development of new tissue.

- AMPK or AMP is the *Activated Protein Kinase.* It is a sensor that is required to balance energy-deprived states by regulating the energy homeostasis and strengthening the backup fuel of the body.

MTOR restricts autophagy because it causes your body to grow, while AMPK enhances autophagy because of the energy-deprived state and exhausting of the internal energy stores. When it is deprived of the nutrients, AMPK begins to prevent cellular growth by suppressing the pathway of Mtorc1, which then causes the body to catabolize its weak parts.

What Can Stop Autophagy

The more exhausted your body is from specific nutrient factors like glucose, amino acids, and calories, the bigger the reason for activating autophagy. Without the relevant requirements, the body doesn't really want to begin recycling its stored energy and bodily tissue. But it will do the same when the right conditions are present.

Both AMPK and Mtor detect the availability of nutrients within the body and your cells will decide whether to stimulate growth or switch into autophagy. It is further determined by the growth factors like insulin and mechanical muscle stimuli.

Here are several things that will by default prevent the development of autophagy-like genes and inhibit autophagy.

- Carbohydrates will prevent autophagy because of high insulin and blood sugar. But you can be catabolic and with inactive Mtor while consuming carbs without protein but you will still restrict autophagy due to the presence of nutrients.

- Proteins and amino acids will reduce the need for stimulating autophagy because the body establishes the presence of nutrients around. You can cut down on your protein to the point of not stimulating muscle protein synthesis and becoming catabolic but you will still restrict autophagy because of taking in protein that awakens MTOR. That is the reason why the restriction of protein isn't an effective process of attempting to boost lifespan or autophagy.

- Extra calories from any macronutrient will restrict autophagy. The high content of carbs, exogenous ketones, and insulin while restricting AMPK. While the rise of insulin isn't very high like taking in fat, it will still have to be directed towards storage hence reducing the desire for the body to support autophagy.

Overall, you can consider autophagy being controlled by the nutrients status inside your cells, how nourished it is, the number of amino acids they get accessed to, and your blood sugar level, when was the last time you ate, and what are your energetic needs at that particular time.

How Long Can You Fast for Autophagy?

Around 48-72 hours of fasting is enough to trigger autophagy. This timeline is probably because that is when you would enter into ketosis and begin to generate ketone bodies.

There are no genuine means of measuring autophagy in humans, but it can be approximating by staring at your glucose ketone index and insulin to glucagon ratio.

- Lower insulin to glucagon ratio results in more

catabolism, gluconeogenesis, fat oxidation, and nutrient deprivation.

- A higher amount of insulin to glucagon ratio results in more anabolism, a higher level of insulin, increased blood sugar, and nutrient storage.

- The glucose ketone index describes an approximated insulin-glucagon ration with a reduced score showing higher ketosis and more AMPK.

How long until autophagy takes place in your body depends on the status of your nutrient in the body as well as the presence of specific nutrients, primarily glucose, ketones, and amino acids.

If you are not taking in a lot of carbs or too much protein every day, then you can expect to switch into autophagy faster than a person who has to burn through those calories first.

The more carbs or protein you consume, the longer you will need to fast before you can get into autophagy. Even taking in a lot of calories that your body requires will boost this buffer zone that requires to be burnt through.

That is the reason why it is better to try mild caloric restriction and avoid going past your maintenance calories if your aim is longevity.

It is going to ensure your body is prepared to switch into

autophagy quickly and you will not need to fast for that period to attain the benefits because fasting for a long time has its negative effects.

Here are some things that can make autophagy to kick in faster:

- Fasting and eating zero calories is the best way of triggering autophagy. It will reduce the level of insulin, Mtor, blood sugar, and deny the liver from amino acids and glucose. But the rise of the body's endogenous ketone bodies will activate chaperone-mediated autophagy, which helps in the reduction of dysfunctional organelles.

- Caloric restriction without fasting can make one experience autophagy faster during extended night fasts. If you are not receiving sufficient amino acids, then you will switch into autophagy faster once you stop eating. But you will not receive it during the day because of eating. Protein reduction will trigger autophagy more than preventing carbs, or fats but it will also predispose the person to a lot of muscle loss. The importance of caloric restriction on autophagy can be attained more effectively using intermittent fasting. Extending the period of fasting, and then eating properly with sufficient protein and other nutrients will offer you deeper autophagy but eliminate the unnecessary muscle loss.

- Exercise and resistance training increase AMPK and hence boost autophagy. Exercising exhausts, the body from glycogen and amino acids, thus building a higher demand for autophagy. The mechanical stimuli still trigger Mtor, which can be said to stop autophagy but the MTOR gets stimulated mainly inside the muscle cells.

You require MTOR to generate muscle and nerve cells but not fat cells or tumors. Instead, you need autophagy inside the liver and brain and not the muscles. Fasting and resistance training is the best mix of acquiring the benefits from both Mtor and autophagy while eliminating the negative side effects when in excess.

In conclusion, how fast you switch to autophagy depends on your personal metabolic status, nutrient status, metabolic conditions, energy requirements, and overall health. A person who is consuming moderate to low carbs and has a lower fasting blood glucose and insulin can expect to stimulate autophagy faster than a person who is consuming hundreds of grams of carbs a day. Similarly, a higher diet of protein also takes a lot of time to get into autophagy.

The only thing that you can bang on is that you need to fast for at least some time to reduce the number of amino acids and glucose within the body. Fasting, in general, is also not advised for underweight people, children, pregnant people and very elderly.

Chapter 2: Why it Matters

Autophagy is a highly controlled process wherein sections of eukaryotic cells are self-digested inside a vacuole and the cellular parts are degraded and recycled. The molecular nature of autophagy was first discovered in budding yeast Saccharomyces cerevisiae as a model structure, functioning in all eukaryotic organisms but not in prokaryotes. Autophagic activity is necessary for the improvement of cellular homeostasis and energy balance.

A lot of evidence relates to malfunctions in autophagic processes to most clinically applicable diseases including neurodegeneration, autoimmunity, cardiovascular disease, and diabetes. The creation of autophagy-focused therapies will rely on an extensive understanding of the benefits, and possible results, of changing autophagic activity.

Different forms of autophagy have been differentiated using the cargo is degraded. The most extensively researched type of autophagy —macro-autophagy reduces huge sizes of the cytoplasm and cellular organelles. Also, the selection of individual substrate classes, cytoplasmic organelles, protein aggregates, and bacteria requires special adaptors that identify the cargo and focuses on the autophagosomes membrane. Other types of autophagy comprise of macroautophagy, which requires the direct surrounding of cytoplasmic material through inward folding of the lysosomal membrane, and chaperone-mediated autophagy (CMA).

Initially defined as a hormonal and starvation response, autophagy plays a huge role in biology, including prevention of genotoxic stress, organelle remodeling, tumor suppression, regulation of immunity, pathogen elimination, maternal DNA inheritance, and cellular sustenance. While autophagy is a degradative channel, it also takes part in biosynthetic and secretory processes. Since autophagy plays a big role in most essential cellular functions. It is not a surprise that autophagic dysfunction is related to multiple forms of human diseases.

Misfolded proteins have a tendency to create insoluble compounds that are dangerous to the cells. To solve this problem, the cells rely on autophagy.

Why autophagy is special, the response depends on the degree of flexibility of autophagosomes size and selection of cargo. Autophagy can support degradation en masse for numerous and different forms of substrates allowing cells to quickly and effectively build up recycled basic building materials in the face of a broad type of nutritional deficiencies. Besides this, autophagy is the only medium that is capable of degrading whole organelles, randomly or in a targeted style. This is a critical procedure for regulating homeostasis in the complex landscape of the eukaryotic cell. This process authenticates a quality control mechanism that is important for counteracting the negative effects of aging. Disrupted autophagy has been shown to cause Parkinson's disease, type 2 diabetes, and other forms of disorder that happen in the elderly. Mutations inside the cell death autophagy genes can result in genetic disease. Interruptions in the autophagic machinery have also been connected to cancer. The types of autophagy have been said to be increased in cancer cells because the tumor microenvironment is hypoxic. Additionally, there is on-going research to create drugs that can deal with autophagy in different diseases.

Autophagy refers to a dynamic, multi-step process that consists of autophagosomes development, depletion of the autophagic substrate, and autolysosome development. The development of autophagosomes, a thin membrane vesicle which surrounds cytosolic components into lysosomes for depletion and recycling, represents autophagy. During the time of autophagy stimulation, the cytoplasmic type of microtubule-related protein 1 light chain LC3 is lapidated and admitted to the autophagosomes. LC3 II, which is the lapidated type of LC3, is connected to the autophagosome membrane, which makes LC3 conversion a must for autophagosome development. The popularly used assay for tracking autophagic flux is the turnover of LCB, which measures the content using autophagic flux. But this method is time-consuming and labor intensive, and the results are usually in different experimental settings and difficult to interpret. Understanding the need for a strong method to highlight autophagic compartments with little straining of endosomes, and lysosomes is a critical approach for tracking autophagy and approximating the autophagic flux in active cells.

Now, let us examine the important benefits of autophagy in detail.

Although "self-eating" may look like a bad idea, it can be a source of youth, and for your cells to regenerate. The phrase "autophagy," is a state for our cells to switch into repair damage and heal. This healing state is stimulated when we need to fight infection, save energy, and repair damage. Read on to discover why autophagy matters in your life.

Autophagy Can Save Your Life

No matter how strange it may appear, autophagy is an ancient process whose primary function is to maintain your life. During moments of severe stress, starvation, infection, this process instantly starts to optimize repair while restricting the damage. The mix of intermittent fasting and autophagy can both starve an infectious intruder of glucose, decrease inflammation so that the immune system has an easier time to take action and correct any damage caused by inflammation and infection.

In other words, animals advanced through autophagy to retain energy and repair damage when energy decreased, but it is also a vital part of the human immune system's ability to fight illness and minimize cancer.

Autophagy Boosts the Rate of Metabolism

Autophagy is a process of removing the trash and replacing the cell parts such as mitochondria. Mitochondria are the cellular engines. They burn fat and build ATP, the fuel of your body. There is a lot of toxic creation in mitochondria that can destroy cells, and breaking them down proactively saves the future wear and tear on your cells. Autophagy in other different parts of the cells saves the whole cell work more efficiently not just burning fuel but also build proteins. Healthier cells work efficiently.

Autophagy Decreases the Rate of Neurodegenerative Diseases

A lot of brain aging diseases take a lot of time to develop because they are the outcome of proteins in and around your brain cells that don't work right. Autophagy assists cells to clean up the proteins that don't do their work and they are less likely to add. For example, autophagy removes amyloid in Alzheimer's disease and a-synuclein in Parkinson's disease. There is an explanation why dementia is believed to be at par with diabetes: the constant high blood sugar controls autophagy from activating, making it difficult to prevent these cells from clutter.

Autophagy Controls Inflammation

Autophagy stimulates a "Goldilocks" degree of inflammation by quelling the immune response you require. Autophagy can boost inflammation when an invader is available by stimulating the immune system to attack. In most cases, autophagy reduces inflammation from your immune response by halting the signals that trigger it.

Autophagy Boosts the Performance of Muscles

As you build microtears and inflame muscles while exercising, the muscles need repair. The demand for energy increases. Your muscle cells will respond to this by getting into autophagy to decrease the energy needed to use the muscle and enhance the balance of energy to lower the risk of future damage.

Autophagy May Enhance the Quality of Life

The advantages of anti-aging may appear to be too good to be true, but the truth is more than the outer layer of the skin. Since the 1950s, scientists have been researching the process of autophagy, but recent studies have disclosed more about how it enhances cellular health. Rather than consuming new nutrients, the cells undergo autophagy to recycle the damaged parts they have, eliminate toxic material and fix themselves up. When your cells repair on their own, they work better, and they can work like younger cells. You may have noticed that some people have a very separate chronological and biological age. The degree of damage a body has taken and how it has managed to repair plays a big role in these differences.

Prevents the Onset of Cancer

Autophagy can inhibit processes that are pro-cancer such as chronic inflammation, genome instability, and DNA damage response. Mice that researchers have genetically made to experience impaired autophagy have increased the speed of cancer. As cancer develops, it may stimulate autophagy to acquire an alternative form of energy or to hide from the immune system, although a lot of research is required. It is still not known the amount of chemotherapy-induced damage to non-cancerous cells stimulates autophagy. In the future, there would be a debate about the amount of destruction chemotherapy does to cancer cells versus our own cells. In the following case, more research is expected.

Autophagy Boosts the Health of the Skin

The cells that you expose to the world experience a lot of damage from air pollution, cold, chemicals, heat, humidity changes, and physical damage. That is the reason why it doesn't appear worse for wear. Once the cells of your skin hold toxins and damage, they start to age in place. Although your body creates new cells, autophagy can assist repair the current ones so that you glow well. Skin cells fight bacteria that may destroy the body, so it is important to support them as they clean the clutter.

Autophagy Enhances Your Digestive Health

The cells inside your gastrointestinal tract are always triggered to function. In fact, a large percentage of your feces are your cells. With the help of autophagy, your digestive cells can repair and restore, clean themselves of junk, and activate the immune system as required. Since a chronic immune system within the gut can exhaust and inflame your bowels, an opportunity to repair, rest and recover is crucial to your health. Stimulate autophagy using a schedule that supports an extended overnight fast and you can offer your gut space it requires to heal.

Fight Infectious Disease

Autophagy can help accept an immune response when required. Next, the process of autophagy can eliminate specific microbes directly from the inside cells like Mycobacterium tuberculosis, or even viruses like HIV. Autophagy can still eliminate the toxins generated by infections, which is necessary for foodborne illness.

Autophagy Can Boost a Healthy Weight

Below are unique benefits of autophagy that create a healthy body:

- Autophagy demands fat-burning to be turned on but spares protein. On a very long fast, you will lose a protein mass, but in short fasting periods, you can stimulate autophagy, spare protein, burn fat, and receive all the benefits of a leaner, and fitter you.

- Autophagy suppresses unnecessary inflammation. Chronic inflammation increases insulin, resulting in more weight storage-and less inflammation assist decrease the percentage of insulin.

- Autophagy decreases toxins inside the cell body. As long as you can remove toxins, they are less likely to require fat cells to store them.

- Autophagy permits metabolic efficiency by repairing the sections of cells that make and package proteins and synthesis energy, which is important when cells require to shift to fat-burning for energy.

It Reduces the Death of Cells

Compared to cell death, the death of a cell is messy and builds garbage to clean up. Your body awakens inflammation to perform the clean –up. The higher the percentage of cells that repair themselves before they are damaged beyond repair, the less effort your body put into cleaning old cells and regenerating new ones. Minimal inflation is involved in regenerating tissues. You can make use of this energy to substitute cells that require continuous renewal such as digestive cells. Although there are specific cells that need to be turned over a lot, not all cells need this. A lot of repair with minimal cleanup is a huge mix of success. While there are a lot of health benefits you can gain, it is a repair response to stress.

As we close on this chapter, autophagy performs two main roles. First, it removes damaging materials and foreign invaders. Secondly, it synthesizes cellular materials for energy during times of starvation. Improper control of autophagy is a big factor for numerous diseases like diabetes, autoimmune diseases, cancer, and infections. Not only does it eliminate damaged materials-it also activates senescence and enhances the cell present antigens on its surface. Researchers have started to establish autophagy as a critical process in both pathology and physiology.

Chapter 3: Autophagy Without Fasting

While fasting for three days stimulates autophagy that enhances longevity and detox. But still, it is possible to activate autophagy without fasting for such a long period.

As previously defined, autophagy is the cellular detoxification process that demands abstinence of nutrients.

Any form of energy whether protein, carbs, fat, exogenous ketones or fiber will restrict autophagy.

To stimulate the autophagy, your liver glycogen has been low, you need to deprive Mtor, which is the channel that causes your cells to grow, and replicates. You have to upregulate AMPK, which is the fuel sensor that is produced when fat burning and energy deprivation happens; and you require to be in this state of depletion for at least a day or even more.

But, autophagy happens in different tissues all the time. There are even certain foods and compounds that enhance autophagy. Even heat saunas and exercise can activate autophagy.

Are You in Autophagy?

Instead of looking at autophagy as something that is controlled by food consider it as regulated by the general energy homeostasis of your body.

Any time your body is in a suppressive condition, you will be burning a lot of fat, keeping your lymph system active, and activating autophagy at least a bit more.

As a result, if you were to improve the AMPK boasting channels that ensure your body burn its endogenous fuel sources and deprives the Mtor boasting channels that record the presence of abundant nutrients, then you can generate mild autophagy while still eating on a normal basis.

Below are some tips for that.

1. Fasting for autophagy

You will still need to practice intermittent fasting each day for some period.

To increase AMPK and autophagy, you want to suppress your liver glycogen, which will result in a lower amount of insulin, deprived Mtor, and high amount of fat oxidation.

There are approximately 100-150 grams of glycogen within the liver, which requires around a day for depletion to happen. At least, you will want to fast for 18-20 hours daily to trigger your body to get into this empty state.

That is the reason why fasting between 16-8 hour fasting window isn't sufficient to increase the growth hormone or attain the benefits of autophagy.

2. Consume a low carb

Any time you eat, you will want to eat relatively low amounts of carb to control lower glycogen stores. Even if you consume a non-ketogenic diet, you don't want to consume more carbs which your body requires because it is going to send a signal to your body that you don't need to burn fat, and you have sufficient energy in the system.

A low carb dieting isn't the end-all-be-all but it is naturally going to cause more regular fasting and low glycogen states, which will increase autophagy.

Muscle glycogen isn't important when it comes to autophagy because muscle glycogen is mainly used for extreme physical exertion. Liver glycogen is the one that controls your blood sugar and detects the general energy homeostasis of your body.

For autophagy, you need to establish lower liver glycogen without worrying about muscle glycogen because muscle glycogen can be suppressed even without consuming carbohydrates.

3. Limit your calories

You don't want to consume high levels of calories or a high percentage of fat because they are going to increase the level of Mtor and overwhelm autophagy. Energy is energy and it is not important where it is originating from.

Caloric restriction can basically boost autophagy to some level. In fact, the restriction of caloric levels enhances longevity and it is one of the less popular methods of doing so.

You don't need to supply your body with excess energy, it doesn't need because it will cut down on its endogenous energy production. Taking more calories that are required of any type can result in disease, oxidative stress, and obesity.

Consuming fewer calories can boost your mitochondrial density, which implies that you will manage to generate more energy with fewer calories. This has a lot of anti-aging advantages and increases your general energy levels.

4. Exercise and autophagy

Aerobic exercise definitely triggers more autophagy because it enhances the lymph flow more so than resistance training. But both are required to maintain a lean mass.

If you were to perform cardio alone at a fasted condition while consuming a caloric deficit diet, then you will activate autophagy but autophagy is a catabolic process that will make you lose lean muscle tissue.

For that reason, if you are consuming lower calories, then it is important to because you will maintain your muscle and is very critical for longevity. You would live longer and healthier if you want to experience less autophagy but maintain muscle instead of becoming skinny fay but more autophagy.

The concept is to trigger AMPK, which notify your body that it has to switch over to burning its energy backup stores.

These foods hold the similarity of increasing fat burning, reducing blood sugar, enhancing anti-oxidants, and stimulating important hermetic effect on your body.

Plants have anti-nutrients that are basically toxins. But in small amounts, they can cause your metabolism to become ant fragile and stimulate additional longevity-boosting metabolic channels like PGC-1, SIRT1, and many more.

5. Low amount of insulin and low Mtor

Suppressing insulin and consuming less protein will prevent the Mtor which can assist improve autophagy. But there is another trade-off when it comes to maintaining the muscle mass.

Excess autophagy can make you catabolic if you remain there for too long. That is why it is better to remain in a semi-autophagy condition most of the time.

Here is a program for gaining the benefits of both autophagy and building muscle.

- Fast every day if you can.

- Eat autophagy stimulating foods like green tea, turmeric, coffee, and others.

- Perform resistance training in a depleted and low glycogen condition to enhance growth hormones.

- After training, take in anabolic amino acids and protein like leucine.

6. Dry fasting autophagy

This is the most extreme way of boosting autophagy. Therefore, theoretically, you can stimulate stem cells and autophagy within just a day of dry fasting.

It may look very extreme and even dangerous but the truth is that mild dehydration can benefit the body through the same procedure of hormesis. The pro-autophagy condition belongs to this part.

You are probably not dehydrated while dry fasting because

burning fatty acids inside the Krebs cycle generates water and hydrogen. Funny enough, you will not stop urinating during dry fasting because you are breaking down your body fat into water.

Dehydration for too long can be dangerous but restricting your water consumption can make you get into autophagy faster.

7. Activate the lymph system

Everything that activates the lymph system will result in a carryover effect to autophagy because of boosting microcirculation.

Sweating through exercise, heat saunas, hot yoga, red light therapy, rebounding and everything that ensures your blood continues to flow at least will assist to flush out toxins inside your body.

You want to sweat well every day, whether through thermal heat, exercise, yoga, or taking spicy foods. This ensures that your detox channels are activated and allow you to use autophagy faster.

Foods that are better for the lymph system consist of teas, coffee, spirulina, medicinal mushrooms, and spicy herbs.

8. Autophagy activation foods

Certain foods trigger autophagy such as green tea, ginger, coffee, ginseng, medicinal mushrooms, elderberries, and berberine.

Autophagy and Exercise

Some of the methods in which exercise enhances autophagy include:

- It induces autophagy inside peripheral tissues and within the brain. Lab mice who are deprived of exercise and starvation prompted autophagy but not basal autophagy cannot run for long distance like a wild-type mouse and don't achieve the benefits of increased glucose intake by muscle. It could also be that the development of new brain cells by exercise is assisted by autophagy.

- Autophagy supports aerobic performance in times of high altitude training. Hypoxia can also activate autophagy and boost blood flow.

- Exercise triggers the AMPK pathway, which excites autophagy. The stimulation of AMPK is also required. AMPK regulates protein synthesis and breaks down pathways.

    AMPK has a major role in skeletal muscle homeostasis.

Additionally, AMPK has been recently proven to be a major controller of skeletal muscle protein turnover. Protein turnover refers to the balance between protein build up and protein breakdown over the course of the day. In case your protein synthesis surpasses the level of the protein's being broken down, then you will be in a more anabolic condition.

Autophagy is crucial to boost skeletal muscle softness in response to exercise endurance.

An exercise that is controlled in a fasted state indicates a huge rise in LC3B-II level compared with a fed state, which shows exercise done during fasting has a better autophagic response.

This is sensible because you will be tapping straight into your body fat for energy rather than burning through the food you ate.

Aerobic exercise and low-intensity cardio burn mainly fat and ketones for fuel, which allow the body to continue generating energy from stored body fat. This offers room for you to continue exercising for a long time without getting into an energy crisis.

Getting more fat adapted through intermittent fasting Consuming a low carb ketogenic diet, and aerobic conditioning will help the body to switch into autophagy quickly.

Both autophagy and the Mtor are important for skeletal muscle homeostasis. In the absence of the anabolic trigger of Mtor, you will not maintain or build muscle. Similarly, without autophagy, you will collect proteins that trigger inflammation.

Autophagy will not enhance the growth of muscle directly but it makes your tissues to become resilient against catabolic stressors that you may experience in times of resistance training.

It is also important for ensuring that the muscles you have are quality and not linked with dysfunctional proteins.

Exercises that boost autophagy-like exercise and fasting boost anabolic hormones and channels that can allow muscles to grow.

But, additional exercise can lead to excessive autophagy activation and this may result in catabolism and muscle atrophy. A lot of energy deprivation prevents recovery and denies anabolic growth.

Anything that is in excess can cause severe effects and result in imbalances. The body yearns for homeostasis and works best when in a balanced state.

How much autophagy is bad relies on your daily anabolic-catabolic balance, which depends on how much you exercise, how many calories you consume, and the amount of fasting you do.

You want to have autophagy stimulated in certain parts like kidneys, brain, heart, and liver. What you don't want is a lot of autophagy in the muscles. However, that is where you want to experience more Mtor.

During resistance training and intermittent fasting, it provides you the best perfect stimulus for Mtor and autophagy in exactly those areas you want them to be.

Resistance Training Builds Your Brain, Detoxes Your Body, and Develops Your Physique

As the name goes, resistance training subjects your muscles up against a force that resists movement. Think of kettlebell training, body weight workouts, and weightlifting. Resistance training is short and intense, causing your muscles to release force from ATP stores rather than depending on oxygen. That short, powerful stress to your body system is important for you.

- Resistance training causes your muscles to become stronger but it also enhances your brain so you move better. In a recent study, 15 men were instructed to lift weights for 14 weeks. At the end of the period, their muscle could produce more force, but the most interesting thing was their neural drive-the ability to push electrical signals from the brain to muscle also became stronger. With a strong neural drive, you experience a precise control of the way you move.

- Resistance training detoxes your body. Keep in mind that your lymphatic system passes through your entire body, nourishing your cells in a clear fluid known as lymph. Lymph accumulates the waste from your cells and clears it, but unlike blood, lymph has no organ to take it through your body. It depends on physical movement. One study discovered that 10-15 minutes of short muscle contractions enhanced the lymph flow by 300-600%.

- Resistance training increases the rate of metabolism, making sure you are in a fat-burning state. It also boosts insulin sensitivity, and the muscle you create will burn fat for you while you rest. This is a three-pronged technique for burning a lot of fat.

- Strength training increases the density of the bone.

- Strength training results in a sharp rise in testosterone and a 200-700% increase in human growth hormone, increasing muscle growth and fat loss in both men and women.

Both resistance training and aerobic exercises are excellent ways to hack your biology, and each offers a special set of benefits. So it is good if you combine them.

Chapter 4: Autophagy and Keto diet

Autophagy is an important process that restores worn-out cells during starvation and fasting. It is a critical aspect of anti-aging and longevity experienced in caloric restriction. Fasting is one of the most effective methods of increasing autophagy.

Ketosis refers to the metabolic state of high ketone utilization and production. It occurs when your body's glycogen stores are suppressed and the liver generates ketones that replace glucose. You can experience ketosis during fasting, or when under a low carb ketogenic diet.

Ketosis and autophagy support each other even though they are not mutually inclusive. Still, you can be in ketosis without autophagy and you can experience autophagy without ketosis. It is only that you will see them together because they share similar principles.

Does Autophagy Need Ketosis

Here's what controls autophagy and ketosis:

- Autophagy is stimulated under energy deprivation caused by a deficiency of amino acid, fasting, thermoregulation, and glucose restriction. In metabolism, you will require little insulin, high AMPK, and low Mtor.

- Ketosis is attained when there is glucose restriction. The main feature that leads to the development of ketone bodies is carbohydrate deficiencies and glycogen depletion. Protein can also lead to carbohydrate synthesis via gluconeogenesis. However, it is secondary and doesn't impact ketosis that much. As a result, you don't need low insulin or low Mtor although it always happens.

You can experience ketosis while consuming high amounts of Mtor and higher insulin because you consumed something that contains high levels of protein. It will regulate nutritional ketosis and high level of ketones but it will inhibit autophagy because of the high nutrient content aspect of Mtor that prevents autophagy.

Autophagy doesn't need ketosis to be stimulated because you can fast for up to 3 days and still not experience ketosis, based on the nature of your keto-adaptation. But remaining in ketosis fulfills most of the prerequisite of autophagy-like low blood glucose, low insulin, and lower Mtor. You only need to base it on the period you have been fasting for.

Measure Ketones to Determine Autophagy

There are no genuine methods to measure autophagy in human beings but it can be estimated by reviewing the glucose ketone index and the ratio of insulin to glucagon.

Lower insulin to glucagon ratio indicates more ketogenesis, fat oxidation, catabolism, and nutrient deprivation.

A higher ratio of insulin to glucagon indicates more anabolism, increased blood sugar, higher insulin and nutrient storage.

The glucose ketone index reveals an estimated ratio of insulin-glucagon with a lower score reflecting higher ketosis and more AMPK.

The time it takes before autophagy starts depends on the nutrient status of your body, and the availability of specific nutrients, especially glucose, and ketones.

If you are not eating a lot of carbs or too much protein daily, then you can expect autophagy to kick in faster than that person who has to burn through those calories first.

Autophagy During Ketosis

The most effective method of stimulating autophagy and ketosis is fast for a few days. This will trigger energy depletion and boost ketone production.

Autophagy is critical for the production of ketone bodies. Mice lacking autophagy have a lower synthesis of ketones by the liver. Gluconeogenesis isn't affected by this, which makes autophagy a necessary part of shifting into ketosis and becoming keto-adapted. Without sufficient autophagy, you will remain more in the sugar burning state.

Ketosis boosts brain macroautophagy by stimulating Sirt. Ketone bodies also activate chaperone-mediated autophagy (CMA), which focuses on certain amino acids and substrates. Beta-hydroxybutyrate and other ketones tend to be high in times of fasting and starvation. However, it also increases when you consume a ketogenic diet.

In nature, your body will get into ketosis during moments when you don't eat well or during winter when there are little carbohydrates and you mainly consume meat. Calorie restriction, protein intake, and limited carbs would ensure that you remain flexible with how quick you activate autophagy and get into ketosis.

Autophagy on Keto

Experiencing ketosis while consuming the ketogenic diet can boost the autophagy process and recycle unique proteins via chaperone-mediated autophagy. This can still happen even while eating as long as your carbs and protein remain low.

A ketogenic diet can limit neuronal injury through autophagy and mitochondrial pathways in seizures. It emulates a lot of features of the fasted physiology like Mtor and lowers insulin.

Specific fats like MCT oil or even coconut oil boost the release of ketone bodies, which enhances ketosis and CMA. But a lot of calories from any macronutrients even fat will still inhibit a fast by elevating Mtor and insulin. That is the reason why the most you can acquire with is 1 tsp of ketone boosting fats during a fast.

However, the ketogenic diet emulates most benefits of fasting and probably helps stimulate autophagy faster than other diets. But for that to succeed, you would require to adhere to the real therapeutic macros of 5% carbs, 70-80% fat, and 15-20% protein. Many people eat a lot of protein and carbs which is better but it's not going to regulate a constant state of autophagy.

While your body can get into ketosis without fasting or autophagy, intermittent fasting is the right way to activate burning fat and keto-adaptation. Consuming the ketogenic diet without fasting may trigger some basal macroautophagy but would occur mainly in between meals.

If you were to compare the health benefits and metabolic effects of the keto diet and fasting-induced autophagy, then fasting would take the first lead. The ketogenic diet helps many tissues like seizures, weight loss, diabetes, and insulin resistance but all are enhanced with extended fasting.

Consuming a low carb ketogenic diet that regulates carbs and doesn't over-do protein is a great basal template for controlling good metabolic health and being ready to get into autophagy faster.

Besides fasting, the therapeutic ketogenic diet that includes some type of intermittent fasting and not more than 2 meals per day is the nearest thing you can get to an autophagy-mimicking diet.

Eating once every day on a keto combined with exercise, consuming autophagic foods, and exposure to other hermetic stressors is one of the most autophagy boosts you can attain while sticking within the 24-hour period. In general, the actual benefits of autophagy start after 24 hours and extend for 3-5 days of fasting.

Are Ketones the Best Fuel for Burning Fat?

If you have ever been to a gas station to pump fuel into your car, you must have seen these three numbers (87-89-93) listed on the pump. But what do they really represent? Maybe someone has ever told you that those numbers represent the rating of something known as octane, which defines the level of compression a fuel can endure before igniting. Higher octane means the less likely the fuel is going to pre-ignite at higher pressures and destroy your engine.

Your body is like a car because it needs fuel to run. Food is your octane, but you can choose the type of fuel to use. You can decide to run on a low octane(sugar) or a high octane(fat). Feeding your body with sugar fuel is likely to cause your body to burst out with fat and be destroyed with chronic disease. On the flip side, fat fuel is highly efficient and will ensure you remain lean.

How Ketones are Generated

Ketones are generated when very little amounts of carbs are consumed and the body breaks down fats. As a result, it produces fatty acids which are burned off within the liver through beta-oxidation. Similar to fats, carbs are one of the major food types. But carbs change into sugar when synthesized by the body, which results in obesity and health challenges. Alternatively, the human brain and body prefer ketones as its main energy source because it runs 70 percent more efficiently than sugar.

From an evolutionary perspective, this preference looks sensible. Keeping in mind that carbs were not easily accessible during prehistoric days.

Why You Need to Make Ketones Your Main Fuel

The state in which the body processes ketones as its major fuel is known as ketosis. Ketones are produced when the body has an insufficient amount of sugar. When the body is deficient of sugar, you switch to ketosis.

Your body needs the energy to control metabolism. This energy is kept as glycogen or fat. Until your body requires energy, glycogen is stored inside the skeletal muscles and liver. When glycogen is stored in your body, it is changed into sugar when needed. Because it is easier for your body to utilize this energy, you have to use it before it starts to burn fat. In the absence of glycogen, your body will convert stored fat into ketones.

A typical human being has around 600 grams of glycogen

inside the body. This is approximately 500 grams in skeletal muscles and 100 grams in the liver.

What Foods to Eat to Produce Ketones

Diet experts have marketed the keto diet because it is effective at burning fat. However, most keto diet resources don't talk about the right foods and nutrients that stimulate cravings. As a result, humans continue to gain weight and grow unhealthy bodies. That is why you need to carefully consider the foods you eat while using ketones to decrease body fat.

It is good to take seafood, pasture-raised eggs, and grass-fed meats because they add protein in your body. Take in carbohydrates from dark green leafy vegetables, and it should make around 5-10% of your diet.

Don't forget to include berries. They are best for low sugar content and high levels of phytonutrients so you should include blackberries, blueberries, and raspberries. Include a serving of berries daily for its excellent antioxidant protection.

Is it Possible to Induce Autophagy Without Starving Yourself?

While fasting is the easiest route to turn off nutrient-sensing pathways, but that is not for everyone as we shall see later. Despite that, most of the physiological responses of a ketogenic diet emulate fasting and the drop in insulin that happens along with the diet is in part responsible. In the animal model, the ketogenic diet has proved to upregulate autophagy inside the brain and demonstrated a drop production of a highly inflammatory molecule, cytochrome C [8].

If conducted well, the ketogenic diet will trigger the metabolic condition of ketosis where blood ketones have been increased. Beta-hydroxybutyrate, the main ketone body, has been found to activate chaperone-mediated autophagy in vitro. But this was in the context of nutrient deprivation.

There is a lot of research that reveals the neuroprotective effects of the ketogenic diet, and the way the diet could substitute the desire for fasting and this could be related to the stimulation of autophagy. For that reason, the ketogenic diet could be used to induce autophagy.

The point here is that ketogenic diet emulates fasting in many ways, and has been proven to induce autophagy in animal models. It is a great alternative to fasting.

Chapter 5: Fast Your Way to Autophagy

Fasting requires that you restrict yourself from consuming calories for a certain period of time. It seems to generate some significant health benefits. Some of these benefits include weight loss, changes to risk factors for diabetes, and heart disease, and a longer lifespan.

Researchers have been attempting to reach to the bottom of why fasting is connected to longevity for years. Lab monkey and mice that fast in the lab studies tend to live longer than those that feed regularly.

Research indicates that minimizing calories turns on genes that cause cells to resent resources. The cells enter a preservation or "famine mode," where they are much more resistant to disease. They also get into a process called autophagy, where the body starts to clean out the old, unwanted, and irrelevant cellular material, plus fixing and recycling damaged sections.

In research where mice fasted for 24-hours, the mice were found to contain a high percentage of autophagosomes, an indication that autophagy is taking place. Now we need to be careful as we link this directly to humans because mouse metabolism is faster than ours.

Although it is difficult to measure autophagy outside the lab environment, professionals say that that the autophagy process is activated after 18-20 hours of fasting in human beings. While the optimal benefits take place between 48-72-hour mark. If this looks overwhelming, remember that intermittent fasting will still provide you with the benefits, but periodically you may consider a longer fast to fully activate autophagy and perform some spring cleaning for your cells. Of course, you need to contact your doctor before you get on any fasting regimen.

Activating autophagy isn't connected to extending longevity, this provides room for researchers to learn more about Alzheimer's and Parkinson's disease. When autophagy doesn't happen frequently, the body gathers different cellular material, including proteins that occur in large amounts in Parkinson's, Alzheimer's and cancer. Researchers believe that extended bouts of autophagy may clear the brain of those extra proteins, and possibly prevent the rise of those diseases.

How to Achieve Autophagy

Although drug companies are trying to develop a pharmaceutical panacea to activate autophagy, and some fitness bloggers say that specific supplements can trigger autophagy—there is only one proven method to activate it: that is fasting. Depriving your body nutrients activates autophagy.

Autophagy stimulation within the body involves two important pathways when the body's nutrients are depleted:

Mtor, or mammalian target of rapamycin, this regulates the nutrients that impact cellular growth, synthesis of protein, and anabolism. It is connected to the stimulation of insulin receptors and new tissue creation.

AMPK or AMP-stimulate protein kinase assists in the maintenance of energy homeostasis and stimulate the body's backup fuel mechanisms.

AMPK and Mtor are accustomed to the presence of nutrients in your body. These two mediums assist your body to decide whether it will stimulate growth response-Mtor-or enter autophagy.

Autophagy still works in concert with two main hormones: insulin and glucagon. People experiencing hypoglycemia or diabetes have challenges controlling, or more sensitive to insulin. When insulin rises, glucagon drops and vice versa. When you fast, you decrease insulin and increase the level of glucagon, which activates autophagy.

How Intermittent Fasting Could Help You Age Slowly

In many areas of our life, lack self-cleaners. There is the self-cleaning oven, and computers can do the same too using automatic virus scans and whatnot. But many other things require time and attention to remove the dirt, grime, and waste that accumulate over time.

Would it be great to have a self-cleaning bathroom? But consider this, what may happen if you fail to regularly maintain our things. That is cars, desks, and kitchens would become dangerous cesspools of dirt, and this would be sickening. That, in one way, is what can occur to our cells. If toxins and waste are not disposed of properly, our cell functions degrade and decline to lead to dull skin, and age-related diseases.

This is exactly what autophagy deals with. Keep in mind that the literal meaning is "self-eating" because your cells will consume their own junk. The result is cleaner, healthier and younger cells.

Let us find out how it works: Our bodies resemble small universes. They consist of trillion of cells, all of which do something in the way we function and how we live. They comprise of different parts that influence those cellular functions. For instance, there are the mitochondria, which produces energy for the cell. The cells also contain proteins, which are necessary for virtually all cellular functions. They give a structure to the cells, perform chemical reactions in the body, and serve as messengers to communicate different types of information across the body.

Although they are microscopic units, each cell plays its role, generating power and products that make your body function properly. These cells perform the work that makes us move, think, and feel everything. These cells grant you the ability to send texts, remember song lyrics, compute mortgage payments, create life-changing memos, and logically reason with toddlers, and everything that you do in your life.

These cells are always working. Most of the time, they do a lot of work, especially when they are young. Everything is new, all systems collectively work together, and things keep plugging along without any hitch. The cells complete their tasks efficiently, and the final result is a young, energized, and healthy body.

That doesn't imply that each cellular system works perfectly throughout. Our usual cellular machinery is damaged with constant use. Many people believe that wear and tear is a normal thing and that no matter what we do, our bodies will break down because of aging. Of course, it is difficult to oppose the natural arc of life and death, but we can slow down the effects of aging. And this is the reason:

Your cells break down its own parts by sequestering them into vacuoles and digesting them. Therefore, they generate waste, especially dead organelles, oxidized particles, and damaged proteins. But unless it is correctly disposed of, that cellular waste remains and builds up in the body, becoming dangerous to our cells. That accumulation is a major factor in the rate of aging. The junk gets in the way and makes everything malfunction. It may appear like jargon from biology class, but the truth is that when the toxins destroy the machinery of your cells, it adds to the aging process. It will cause your skin to appear older, your body to slow, your energy to drop, and your hormones to go haywire.

That is the reason autophagy is critical. When it is functioning well, it is a form of self-renewal, breaking down older structures so that new ones can be developed in their place. The result is that the newer, youthful structures cause our cells to work like they are newer and youthful.

You can imagine how that works out in your daily life. More youthful cells mean softer and healthier skin, faster metabolism, and less fatigue. It implies that your cell universe generates youthfulness everywhere, from your brains, organs to muscles.

In a study conducted in the Journal of Diabetes and Metabolism, the authors describe autophagy as a "survival strategy," which makes more sense. If you consider it from a cellular perspective, it is a survival mechanism. However, from a lifestyle perspective, the technique to survive becomes a strategy to thrive because younger cells mean a younger self.

The Autophagy On/Off Switch

Autophagy is like everything else in our body. As we start to grow old, it naturally declines and loses its efficiency. This means that you are now saddled with a twofold challenge. Your cells collect a lot of junk and your body can't keep up with clearing away the junk because of the frequent exposure to Accelerated Agers. More waste results in more damage. More damage, without a means to fix it, leads to increased aging.

All the cellular waste is connected not only to things like skin damage, but also cancer and neurodegenerative diseases. This drop in autophagy is said to be a critical effect of aging. It is not just the destruction of our cells that is so bad, but also the decline in our ability to correct it.

Another important aspect to consider: Autophagy cannot always be on high. Cells cannot be cleaning waste all the time. They also have to play the role of producing waste. Take it this way: Imagine your kitchen. Let us say you prepare dinner and clean up after the meal. This multistep process involves meal preparation and eliminating waste after you consume.

Therefore, autophagy is a sequence of steps that frees your cellular kitchen of any clutter, and you need all of it to work. In case there is a pileup at the sink, there will be clutter somewhere.

But the catch is that you cannot always in the cleaning mode, you must at least have something to clean up. You need the kitchen to prepare your food, just like in the way your cells need to do other tasks. So when a kitchen is humming, it's a balance between preparing food and cleaning dirt. Typically, that is the same process for your body cells-generating energy to your entire body and then cleaning up the waste products. This is the concept behind autophagy being switched on and off. When the kitchen is getting cleaned, in response to that stressor, autophagy continues to work at its best level keeping in mind the stress response mode. And when you are preparing and eating dinner, autophagy will be at its lowest point. Think of it as electricity. If you connect a lamp, the electricity is always flowing regardless of whether the switch is on or off, but a lot of electricity is required to power it on.

There are two approaches to turn autophagy on and off to prevent aging. First, by naturally inducing stress on your body; and secondly integrate autophagy-activating nutrients.

Advanced Autophagy: The Missing Link in Anti-Aging

Autophagy is the most important breakthroughs in the science of aging. While scientists have been learning this process since the 1950s, only in recent years that we have started to see the effects of stimulating autophagy to enhance the health of our cells. Research released in the Journal of Clinical and Experimental Pathology says that "autophagy boosts cell maintenance by eliminating accumulated toxic waste and using recycled parts as an alternative nutrient resource." This means that autophagy supports longevity because an organism can recover fast from stress-induced cellular damage. As you can expect, when the cells can clean up the damage that they generate, that implies that they can function better. Practically, that means all your body's cells will work better.

Water Fasting

Fasting, a technique of restricting food intake has been used for quite some time.

Water fasting is a form of fast that deprives the body everything except water. It is more popular in recent years as a quick means to lose weight.

Research shows that water fasting could have different health benefits. It may reduce the risk of certain chronic diseases and may trigger autophagy, a process that allows your body to break down and recycle old parts of your cells.

That said, there are limited studies on water fasting. It also comes with several health risks and is not perfect for everyone.

As defined, water fasting is one where you cannot take anything besides water.

Most of the water fasts last between 24-72 hours. But you should not follow water fast for a longer period than this without medical supervision.

Some of the reasons why people attempt water fasting include:

- To lose weight
- Spiritual reasons
- For health benefits
- To get ready for a medical procedure

The major reason why people attempt water fasting is because of the health benefits.

That is because different studies have proven water fasting to provide health benefits. This includes a reduced risk of cancers, diabetes and heart disease.

Water fasting may still improve autophagy. Popular diets like lemon detox cleanse are designed after the water fasting. The lemon detox cleanses only allows you to consume a composition of lemon juice, maple syrup, water, and cayenne pepper, different times per day for up to 7 days.

Despite this, water fasting has different risks and can be very dangerous if followed for a long period.

How Can You Water Fast?

There are no scientific instructions on how you can begin to water fast, but there is a category of people that should not water fast without a medical examination.

This includes people with diabetes, eating disorders, gout, pregnant women, and older adults.

If you have never water fasted before, it is a great idea to spend 3-4 days getting ready to stay without food.

You can do this by taking little portions at each meal or by fasting for part of the day.

While water fasting, you are not allowed to drink or eat anything apart from water.

Many people take 2-3 liters of water per day of a water fast. The water fast lasts between 24-72 hours. You should never water fast for longer than this without medical examination because of the health challenges.

Some people may feel weak during a water fast and may want to avoid running heavy machinery and driving to avoid causing an accident.

How You Can Lose Weight Through Intermittent Fasting

There are different ways in which you can lose weight.

Intermittent fasting is one of the popular ways that people use to lose weight. It is a style of eating that involves daily short-term fasts.

Fasting for a short period allows people to eat consume fewer calories and also improves hormones that control weight.

The three popular methods of intermittent fasting include:

1. The 16/8 Method: This requires a person to skip breakfast daily and eat during an 8-hour feeding window like between 12 noon to 8 pm.

2. Eat-Stop-Eat. In this method, you do one or two 24-hour fasts every week.

3. The 5:2 Diet

The main reason why intermittent fasting helps an individual lose weight is that a person consumes fewer calories.

All the different protocols require a person to skip meals during the period of fasting. Unless you replace it by consuming more while eating, then you will be taking little calories.

A 2014 review study revealed how intermittent fasting has a

significant impact on weight loss. For instance, this study discovered that people who practiced intermittent fasting said to have lost about 0.55 pounds per week.

Additionally, people reported losing 4-7% of their waist circumference.

These are great results, and they show that intermittent fasting can be beneficial to weight loss.

That said, the importance of intermittent fasting is beyond weight loss. It has also other benefits, and may even alleviate chronic disease and expand lifespan.

While counting calorie isn't necessary when performing intermittent fasting, weight loss is highly mediated by a general reduction in calorie consumption.

Intermittent Fasting Can Help You Retain Muscle While Dieting

The worst thing about dieting is that the body tends to exhaust the muscle.

Several studies show that intermittent fasting may be necessary to retain muscle mass.

Take for instance the calorie restriction studies, 25% of the weight loss represented the muscle mass.

Which Fasting is Best for You?

Fasting is a popular trend not just because of the powerful results, but because of many other health benefits that extend from mental clarity to enhanced metabolic risk factors.

So which fasting approach is best for you?

So far you have learned about water fasting and intermittent fasting, but there are still other methods of fasting that you need to know.

First, let us briefly explore 4 other methods before making a final note on the best method of fasting.

Alternate Day Fasting (ADF)

This is a branch of intermittent fasting where individuals restrict all calories for a whole day, the "fast day" followed by a "feed day". In a study that compared ADF to basic caloric restriction discovered that ADF is safe and comparable to caloric restriction in weight loss.

Additionally, research reveals ADF positively support metabolic disorders and several risk factors. And the effects may not be short-term, until 24 weeks after involving ADF. Also, people who have tried ADF consider its diet easier to stick to compared to other types of fasting because there is no eating to tempt you on fast.

Caloric Restriction

For those who doubt whether fasting will produce the necessary results, caloric restriction is a better choice. In 1935, researchers realized that limiting the amount of calorie intake in lab mice extended their lives. The same effect was illustrated in other organisms like fruit flies, worms, and rodents. Studies have gone further to explore the same effect in humans. To take advantage of the benefits, humans must learn to restrict their calorie intake by 40-60%.

Multi-Day Fasts

If you approved by a doctor to fast, you can try multi-day fast. Multi-day fasting for three days with 0-200 calories per day decreased the level of white blood cell counts and allowed the immune system to release new white blood cells.

Fasting-Mimicking Diet (FMD)

For those who are unable to fast without taking any food, this fasting method may be the best for you. Fasting-Mimicking Diet makes the body think it is fasting while you still take food. A normal FMD lasts approximately five days and focuses on balancing protein, carbs, and calories. Members consume around 40% of normal calorie.

Whichever method you select; studies show the health benefits are more than the challenges of feeling hungry.

Chapter 6: The 3-Day Fix to Change your Metabolism

When you have a slower-than-normal metabolism, builds a cascade of negative side effects, this includes mood swings, fatigue, food cravings, and challenges losing weight.

Fortunately, slow metabolism isn't permanent, and with the correct changes to your lifestyle and diet, you can boost your metabolism-and get back to feeling well in the process.

And the best thing is that it doesn't take long to make it happen. With the help of this three-day fix, you will get your metabolism in the right track and reap the benefits of a rising metabolic rate.

Day1: Saturday

Make sure you sleep for 8 hours.

If you had a late night on Friday, use the Saturday morning to catch up on some ZZZ's.

When you fail to have enough sleep, this can affect the hormone balances in the body, which may slow down your metabolism and increase your risk for weight gain.

Lack of sleep is interpreted by the body as an extra stressor. For that reason, cortisol increases, and testosterone decreases.

Purpose to sleep at least 8 hours per night, and ensure those 8 hours involve total sleep without interruptions. The point is that you need to get the high quality sleep that rejuvenates the brain, and restores the body.

What to Eat

Don't miss breakfast.

You may be tempted to skip breakfast, but if you want to maintain your metabolism, find time to take breakfast. A 2018 study found that taking breakfast before going to work out boosts your metabolism post-workout.

And remember to take Greek yogurt. This will balance your gut bacteria and boost the rate of metabolism. To confirm that you are taking the correct gut-balance microorganisms with your breakfast, ensure your Greek yogurt is written, "contains active cultures" on the packaging.

What to Do

If you want to kick start your metabolism, the best way is to perform strength training workouts. Muscle building increases your metabolic rate for up to 2 hours after every 20-minute session.

By performing a strength routine, you will build more muscle, and the more muscle you have, the better the metabolism you will experience.

When to Go to Sleep

You may be tempted to stay up late and catch up with your favorite Netflix queue, but try to fight that urge. If you want to maintain a high metabolism, then you need to get at least 8 hours of sleep-so to make sure you rest to bed before midnight.

Day 2: Sunday

If you sleep before midnight, then you need to wake up around 8 a.m. This provides you with sufficient time to sleep for a healthy metabolism but early enough so that you don't get frustrated when your alarm goes off for work the next day.

What to Drink

Begin your day by taking a cup of coffee.

A little bit of caffeine is enough to boost your metabolism.

Not a coffee person? Don't worry you can get the same effect with a cup of green tea.

And ensure you take enough water.

Research shows that taking 16.9 ounces of water increases the rate of metabolism by 30 percent for 30-40 minutes. This means if you want to make the most from metabolism, then you have to take 16.9 ounces of water different times throughout the day.

What to Do

Prep meals for the week, and make sure to add some chili peppers.

The best ways to prepare for success during the week is to prepare meals on Sundays. And if you would like your meals to boost your metabolism then you need to increase the heat and add some chili peppers into your recipes.

Chili peppers contain a compound called capsaicin that is considered to boost the rate of metabolism.

Boost Your Neat

There is so much that you can do while at the gym to boost your metabolism, but it is what you do outside the gym that has the most impact. So you should try to move a lot in your daily life.

Day 3: Monday

Wake up once you have slept for 8 hours.

Keep in mind that it is a Monday, which means you resume going to work and you will have less flexibility in your wakeup time.

If you need to wake up early, ensure you adjust your time of going to sleep on Sunday to ensure that you get a full 8-hour sleep for enhancing the benefits of metabolism.

What to Eat

Include some protein to each meal.

If you want to use your diet to boost your metabolism, focus on adding protein to every meal.

Adding lean protein like chicken, eggs, and dairy to your diet will boost your metabolism in two ways. First, it will assist muscle growth, and muscle holds up plus the foods are challenging for your body to digest, so it requires a lot of energy from your body to absorb them than other foods.

What to Do

Stress slows down the rate of metabolism. If you want to remove stress, meditation is a great way to keep stress at bay. Mindfulness meditation has been found to reduce the percentage of cortisol, and you can experience the benefits with as little as 10-15 minutes of meditation training per day.

What You Should Do the Entire Week

This three-day fix is a great start to elevate your metabolism – but it is just the beginning.

A healthy metabolism will maintain your body shape and increase your energy levels. If you want to lose weight, increasing your metabolic rate means you will begin to see the benefits early.

So don't just make it a weekend fix. Aim to make permanent changes in your life so that your metabolism can be constantly at its peak.

For the remaining days of the week and your entire life

1. Focus on getting 8-hour high-quality sleep per night.

2. Consume a lot of protein with each meal.

3. Meditate daily to reduce stress.

4. Remain hydrated

5. Consume probiotic-rich foods

6. Take at least three metabolism-boosting workouts per week.

However, if you want to experience the real permanent changes to your metabolism, you will need to commit to real, lasting changes in your lifestyle and diet.

Autophagy Conclusion

Autophagy is not easy as we would like it to be, but with the current knowledge of how it is stimulated, there are lifestyle practices that at least wouldn't hurt to attempt. The caution to all this is that we don't want these processes to be on or off all the times and we certainly don't want to be in a catabolic state.

The growth factors that restrict autophagy also allow us to increase muscle mass, heal wounds, and control many cellular processes for growth and development. It is also important to realize that most of the research done in animal models and based on practical implementation, not all data is directly applicable to humans.

We still acknowledge that autophagy can play a big role in the prevention and control of many age-related diseases and that learning how to activate autophagy is an important tool in our toolbox, just like how we think of the ketogenic diet.

All in all, autophagy is a very important cellular process that is absolutely needed for the health of our cells and should be given serious attention as we grow old.

Hopefully, this book breaks down everything you wanted to know about autophagy, and now you know how to unlock your body's natural cellular repair code for weight loss, anti-aging, health, and revitalization benefits.

www.ingramcontent.com/pod-product-compliance
Lightning Source LLC
Chambersburg PA
CBHW072108280526
45788CB00006B/2452